Table of Contents

Introduction

Dr. Irwin Stillman practiced as a family physician in Brooklyn, New York, and developed the Stillman Diet in the 1960s. He subsequently wrote a book titled "The Doctor's Quick Weight Loss Diet," and the diet soon became known by the book's title rather than as the Stillman Diet. He later developed variations on the diet, including one that incorporated exercise and another for teenagers that added limited carbohydrates; but the original Stillman Diet is a straightforward high-protein, low-carbohydrate and low-fat diet.

The Stillman Diet was designed by Dr. Irwin Maxwell Stillman in 1967. Also known as Doctor's Quick Weight Loss Diet, named after the book written by Dr. Stillman, it is a low-carb high-protein diet. In fact, rumor has it that Dr. Stillman tried this diet himself and lost 50 pounds in just a few weeks. This made him confident about this diet plan, and he started recommending it to obese patients.

The reason it works is it allows you to eat 6 meals per day instead of 3 big meals. This keeps your cells active and metabolism firing. You drink 8 glasses of water per day, so your cells will be hydrated and perform their functions properly. It will also help to flush out the toxins. When you are on this diet, you will mostly consume protein, a moderate amount of fat, and less than a moderate amount of carbs. Carbs get broken down into sugar in the body. And when in excess, they get stored as fat. When your body is on a low-carb diet, it starts using protein as an alternative source of energy. This, in turn, results in weight loss. The Stillman Diet is divided into two phases – Phase 1 and Phase 2. Each phase has different diet requirements, and you need to follow them strictly to lose weight.

Stillman Diet Chart – Phase 1

Stillman Diet Foods To Eat – Phase 1

Proteins – Chicken breast, fish, veal, lean cuts of beef, eggs, and turkey.

Beverages – Black coffee, green tea, black tea, oolong tea, white tea, and water.

Others – Herbs, spices, salt, pepper, and tabasco sauce.

Stillman Diet Foods To Avoid – Phase 1

Vegetables, fruits, alcohol, condiments, bread, butter, oil, rice, pasta, aerated drinks, and artificially sweetened drinks.

Stillman Diet Supplements – Phase 1

Consult your doctor or dietitian to know if you need to take supplements while you are on this diet. Typically, you may take vitamin and mineral supplements every two days to support your body and reduce the risk of falling ill.

Stillman Diet Workout Plan – Phase 1

For Phase 1, stick to stretching, meditation, and yoga. Avoid going to the gym, running, or any other rigorous form of exercise. Here is what you can do.

Neck rotations – 1 set of 10 reps

Shoulder rotations – 1 set of 10 reps

Arm circles – 1 set of 10 reps

Wrist rotations – 1 set of 10 reps

Waist rotations – 1 set of 10 reps

Ankle rotation – 1 set of 10 reps

Yoga or meditation

Stretch

How You Will Feel After Stillman Diet Phase 1

After completing the first week of Stillman Diet, you will lose a lot of water weight. You will kickstart your metabolism, mobilize the fat, and build lean muscle mass. You may feel weak and experience mood swings as you will be on a low-carb diet. You might also feel tired and fatigued all the time. To prevent this, you should do yoga/meditation and stretching exercises. But, you will look forward to the next week as you will move on to the next phase, which allows you to reintroduce carbs into your diet.

Stillman Diet Chart – Phase 2

Stillman Diet Foods To Eat – Phase 2

Protein – Fish, chicken breast, mushroom, egg, lean cuts of beef, turkey, duck, and veal.

Veggies – All veggies but in minimum quantities.

Fruits – Peach, grapes, pluot, plum, guava, apple, pear, orange, lemon, grapefruit, watermelon, and muskmelon.

Beverages – Green tea, black tea, oolong tea, white tea, and black coffee.

Others – Herbs, spices, salt, pepper, and tabasco sauce.

Stillman Diet Foods To Avoid – Phase 2

Fruits – Mango, banana, and jackfruit.

Dairy – Full-fat cream, milk, and yogurt.

Beverages – Soda, packaged fruit juice, and alcohol.

Stillman Diet Supplements – Phase 2

You would be eating more nutritious foods as compared to Phase 1, but even then, if you feel weak; consult your doctor to know if you should take supplements.

Stillman Diet Workout Plan – Phase 2

During the Phase 2 of the Stillman diet, you can follow the below workout regimen.

Neck rotations – 1 set of 10 reps

Shoulder rotations – 1 set of 10 reps

Arm circles – 1 set of 10 reps

Wrist rotations – 1 set of 10 reps

Waist rotations – 1 set of 10 reps

Ankle rotation – 1 set of 10 reps

Jumping jacks – 1 set of 10 reps

Mountain climbers – 1 set of 10 reps

Scissor kicks – 1 set of 10 reps

Yoga/ meditation

Stretch

How You Will Feel After Stillman Diet Phase 2

By the end of Phase 2, you will look slimmer, weigh lesser, and your confidence levels will soar high.

Following a good lifestyle rewards you with both physical and mental strength. And you will love your new self! Now, the big question is, how much weight can you expect to lose? Here's your answer.

Other Foods To Eat

Stillman Diet - Other Foods To Eat

With so much stress on including only proteins in your daily diet, you must be wondering what exactly you are allowed to eat. The diet recommends the inclusion of some crucial food items. You can safely eat protein-rich food to your heart's content. Such foods include low-fat cheese, lean meat, soft or hard-boiled eggs, farmer's cheese, lean fish like flounder, cod, haddock, low-calorie gelatin, and other food such as lobsters, crabs, shrimps, and oysters.

In the next section, we list out other foods you should avoid when you are on the Stillman diet.

Other Foods To Avoid

Stillman Diet - Other Foods To Avoid

1. Foods That Add Flavor

The Stillman diet recommends banishing fat and carb-rich food, such as salad dressings, mayonnaise, ketchup, and other similar foods that are used for adding flavor to the dishes. However, the use of spices and herbs to add more flavors to the meal is allowed.

2. Fat-Rich Foods

The diet eliminates all fatty food such as margarine, dense skin poultry, greasy, fried foods, whole-fat dairy products, sauce, gravy, tartar, etc.

3. All Types of Sugar

All types of sugars, natural or refined, are restricted during this diet. Except for brown sugar, molasses, white sugar, corn syrup, sugar cane syrup, natural sugar and different varieties of refined sugars, such as candy sugar, fruit juices, syrup with sweeteners, sweet desserts, etc., are a big NO in this diet's blueprint.

4. Starchy Foods

Foods that are rich in starch, including whole wheat, legumes, dried potatoes, white bread, barley, etc., are banished from this diet.

5. Vegetables and Fruits

The Stillman diet plan also banishes the consumption of vegetables and fruits. Lettuce and salad too are struck off your daily diet, which may bring a smile on the face of many!

So, what if you continue to avoid eating veggies, fruits, and other nutritious foods? In the next section, we will discuss the adverse effects of following this diet.

Stillman Diet Side Effects

Here are the side effects of following the Stillman diet for too long without the supervision of a professional.

- Malnutrition
- Digestion problems
- Fatigue and muscle pain
- Weak bones
- Kidney stones
- High cholesterol levels in the blood
- Short-term weight loss

This diet is for those who are looking for a quick weight loss plan for an upcoming event or just to kickstart their fat mobilization. Do not follow this diet plan if your doctor or dietitian doesn't approve of it. Also, take a break of at least 2 weeks before following this diet plan again.

Recipes

Keto Beef Egg Roll Slaw

Recipe Summary

prep: 15 mins

cook: 15 mins

total: 30 mins

Servings: 6

Yield: 6 servings

Ingredients

2 tablespoons sesame oil

½ cup diced onion

5 green onions, chopped, white and green parts separated

3 cloves garlic, minced

1 ½ pounds ground beef

1 tablespoon chili-garlic sauce (such as sriracha)

½ teaspoon ground ginger

sea salt to taste

ground black pepper to taste

1 (14 ounce) package coleslaw mix

3 tablespoons soy sauce

1 tablespoon apple cider vinegar

Directions

Instructions

Step 1

Heat oil in a large skillet over medium-high heat. Add diced onion, white parts of the green onions, and garlic. Saute until onions are translucent and garlic is fragrant, about 5 minutes. Add ground beef, sriracha, ginger, salt, and black pepper. Saute until beef is browned and crumbly, about 5 minutes.

Step 2

Stir coleslaw mix, soy sauce, and cider vinegar into the beef mixture. Saute until coleslaw is tender, about 4 minutes more. Top with the rest of the green onions.

Cook's Note:

Feel free to substitute olive oil for the sesame oil.

Nutrition Facts

Per Serving:

350 calories; protein 20.6g; carbohydrates 12g; fat 24g; cholesterol 74.9mg; sodium 694.1mg.

Mongolian Beef

Recipe Summary

prep: 20 mins

cook: 10 mins

additional: 1 hr 50 mins

total: 2 hrs 20 mins

Servings: 6

Yield: 6 servings

Ingredients

1 pound flank steak

¼ cup chicken stock

1 ½ tablespoons cornstarch

3 tablespoons hot chili oil

2 tablespoons hoisin sauce

1 tablespoon oyster sauce

1 tablespoon dry sherry

2 teaspoons sugar

2 teaspoons soy sauce

2 teaspoons crushed red pepper flakes

2 tablespoons peanut oil

2 tablespoons chopped garlic

1 bunch Swiss chard - rinsed, stems removed and cut into 1/2 inch slices

2 green onions, cut into thin slivers about 2 inches long

1 teaspoon salt

¼ teaspoon black pepper

Directions

Instructions

Step 1

Spread the flank steak out flat, cover with plastic wrap, and place in the freezer until partially frozen, 20 to 30 minutes.

Step 2

Remove beef from the freezer and slice across the grain into very thin slices.

Step 3

Whisk the chicken stock and cornstarch in a freezer-safe bowl until smooth; whisk in the hot chili oil, hoisin sauce, oyster sauce, sherry, sugar, soy sauce, and crushed red pepper flakes. Place the beef into the sauce, stir to coat well. Cover and freeze until frozen, about 1 hour.

Step 4

Remove from the freezer and allow to defrost, about 30 minutes.

Step 5

Heat a wok over high heat until very hot, and pour in the peanut oil. Immediately add garlic, cook and stir in the hot oil until fragrant, about 15 seconds. Mix in the Swiss chard and green onions; cook and stir the vegetables until they turn bright green, about 3 minutes, and then remove from the wok.

Step 6

Pour the defrosted beef mixture into the hot wok; cook and stir until the meat browns and the sauce forms a glaze, 3 to 5 minutes. Return the cooked vegetables to the wok, sprinkle with salt and pepper, mix to combine well; serve hot.

Nutrition Facts

Per Serving:

197 calories; protein 10.6g; carbohydrates 9.5g; fat 13.2g; cholesterol 18.3mg; sodium 707.4mg.

Slow Cooker Chicken Taco Soup

Recipe Summary

prep: 15 mins

cook: 7 hrs

total: 7 hrs 15 mins

Servings: 8

Yield: 8 Servings

Ingredients

1 onion, chopped

1 (16 ounce) can chili beans

1 (15 ounce) can black beans

1 (15 ounce) can whole kernel corn, drained

1 (8 ounce) can tomato sauce

1 (12 fluid ounce) can or bottle beer

2 (10 ounce) cans diced tomatoes with green chilies, undrained

1 (1.25 ounce) package taco seasoning

3 whole skinless, boneless chicken breasts

1 (8 ounce) package shredded Cheddar cheese (Optional)

1 (8 ounce) container sour cream

1 cup crushed tortilla chips

Directions

Instructions

Step 1

Place the onion, chili beans, black beans, corn, tomato sauce, beer, and diced tomatoes in a slow cooker. Add taco seasoning, and stir to blend. Lay chicken breasts on top of the mixture, pressing down slightly until just covered by the other ingredients. Set slow cooker for low heat, cover, and cook for 5 hours.

Step 2

Remove chicken breasts from the soup, and allow to cool long enough to be handled. Stir the shredded chicken back into the soup, and continue cooking for 2 hours. Serve topped with shredded Cheddar cheese, a dollop of sour cream, and crushed tortilla chips, if desired.

Nutrition Facts

Per Serving:

434 calories; protein 27.2g; carbohydrates 42.3g; fat 17.7g; cholesterol 67.8mg; sodium 1596.8mg.

Loaded Cauliflower

Recipe Summary

prep: 10 mins

cook: 45 mins

total: 55 mins

Servings: 4

Yield: 4 servings

Ingredients

1 head cauliflower

½ cup sour cream

½ cup shredded Cheddar cheese

1 teaspoon dry ranch salad dressing mix (such as Hidden Valley Ranch®)

½ teaspoon onion powder

½ teaspoon garlic powder

1 tablespoon butter, cut into small pieces, or more to taste

Directions

Instructions

Step 1

Preheat oven to 350 degrees F (175 degrees C).

Step 2

Place a steamer insert into a saucepan and fill with water to just below the bottom of the steamer. Bring water to a boil. Add cauliflower, cover, and steam until very tender, 15 to 20 minutes. Transfer cauliflower to a bowl, mash, and strain excess water.

Step 3

Mix cauliflower, sour cream, Cheddar cheese, ranch dressing mix, onion powder, and garlic powder together in a 9-inch baking dish; top with butter.

Step 4

Bake in the preheated oven until bubbling, 30 to 45 minutes.

Nutrition Facts

Per Serving:

196 calories; protein 8.2g; carbohydrates 9.8g; fat 14.8g; cholesterol 38.4mg; sodium 226.9mg.

Chinese Barbeque Pork (Char Siu)

Recipe Summary

prep: 10 mins

cook: 2 hrs

additional: 3 hrs

total: 5 hrs 10 mins

Servings: 6

Yield: 6 servings

Ingredients

⅔ cup soy sauce

½ cup honey

½ cup Chinese rice wine (or sake or dry sherry)

⅓ cup hoisin sauce

⅓ cup ketchup

⅓ cup brown sugar

4 cloves garlic, crushed

1 teaspoon Chinese five-spice powder

½ teaspoon freshly ground black pepper

¼ teaspoon cayenne pepper

⅛ teaspoon pink curing salt (Optional)

1 (3 pound) boneless pork butt (shoulder)

1 teaspoon red food coloring, or as desired (Optional)

1 teaspoon kosher salt, or to taste

Directions

Instructions

Step 1

Place soy sauce, honey, rice wine, hoisin sauce, ketchup, brown sugar, garlic, five-spice powder, black pepper, cayenne pepper, and curing salt in a saucepan. Bring to a boil on high heat; reduce heat to medium-high. Cook for 1 minute. Remove from heat. Cool to room temperature.

Step 2

Cut pork roast in half lengthwise. Cut each half again lengthwise forming 4 long, thick pieces of pork.

Step 3

Transfer cooled sauce to a large mixing bowl. Stir in red food coloring. Place pork sections into sauce and coat each piece. Cover with plastic wrap and refrigerate 4 to 12 hours.

Step 4

Preheat grill for medium heat, 275 to 300 degrees F (135 to 150 degrees C) and lightly oil the grate. Line a baking sheet with parchment paper.

Step 5

Remove sections of pork from marinade and let excess drip off. Place on prepared baking sheet. Sprinkle with kosher salt to taste.

Step 6

Transfer pork sections to grate over indirect heat on prepared grill. Cover and cook about 45 minutes. Brush with marinade; turn. Continue cooking until an instant-read thermometer inserted into the center reads 185 and 190 degrees F, about 1 hour and 15 minutes more. Do not use any more marinade on cooked meat until after you boil it.

Step 7

Place leftover marinade in saucepan; bring to a boil; let simmer 1 minutes. Remove from heat. Now you can use it to brush over the cooked pork.

Chef's Notes:

If you happen to be using your standard, backyard kettle-shaped grill, push all your coals to one side, and place your meat on the other. To add an extra layer of protection, you can also put it in a roasting pan, and place that on the grill. Or, forget the great outdoors, and simply roast it in the oven. The only catch is, you'll need to place it under the broiler at the end, to simulate the caramelization we get on the barbeque.

Nutrition Facts

Per Serving:

513 calories; protein 26g; carbohydrates 49.1g; fat 21.9g; cholesterol 89.8mg; sodium 2421.1mg.

Turkey with Dumplings Soup

Recipe Summary

prep: 20 mins

cook: 1 hr 5 mins

total: 1 hr 25 mins

Servings: 10

Yield: 10 servings

Ingredients

½ cup butter, cubed

8 medium carrots, cut into 1-inch chunks

4 stalks celery, cut into 1-inch chunks

1 cup chopped onion

4 ⅔ cups water, divided

2 (10.5 ounce) cans condensed beef consomme

2 teaspoons salt

¼ teaspoon ground black pepper

3 cups cubed cooked turkey

2 cups frozen cut green beans

½ cup all-purpose flour

2 teaspoons Worcestershire sauce

Dumplings:

1 ½ cups all-purpose flour

2 teaspoons baking powder

1 teaspoon salt

2 tablespoons minced parsley

⅛ teaspoon poultry seasoning

¾ cup 2% milk

1 egg

Directions

Instructions

Step 1

Melt butter in a Dutch oven over medium-high heat. Saute carrots, celery, and onion for 10 minutes. Add 4 cups water, consomme, salt, and pepper. Bring to a boil. Reduce heat to low and cover. Cook until vegetables are tender, about 15 minutes.

Step 2

Add turkey and beans to the vegetables. Cook for 5 minutes. Mix flour and Worcestershire sauce with remaining water in a bowl until smooth; stir into turkey mixture. Increase heat and bring to a boil. Reduce heat, cover, and simmer soup until thickened, about 5 minutes.

Step 3

For the dumplings, combine flour, baking powder, and salt in a large bowl. Stir in parsley and poultry seasoning. Combine milk and egg in a separate bowl; stir into flour mixture until just moistened. Drop mixture by tablespoons onto the simmering soup. Cover and simmer until a toothpick inserted into a dumpling comes out clean, about 20 minutes.

Cook's Notes:

May use 2 cups of leftover turkey stock/broth instead of beef broth. Substitute green beans with peas if desired.

Nutrition Facts

Per Serving:

303 calories; protein 18g; carbohydrates 28.8g; fat 12.7g; cholesterol 76.4mg; sodium 1161.4mg.

Gourmet Gouda Turkey Burgers

Recipe Summary

prep: 20 mins

cook: 10 mins

total: 30 mins

Servings: 4

Yield: 4 burgers

Ingredients

1 egg

¼ cup minced onion

1 pound ground turkey

½ cup fine Italian bread crumbs

2 teaspoons liquid smoke flavoring

2 tablespoons Worcestershire sauce

½ teaspoon salt

½ teaspoon ground black pepper

¼ cup panko bread crumbs

1 large portobello mushroom cap, cut into thick slices

1 tablespoon olive oil for brushing

4 ounces Canadian-style bacon

4 ounces sliced Gouda cheese

4 hamburger buns, split and toasted

¼ cup spicy brown mustard, or to taste

½ cup mayonnaise, or to taste

Directions

Instructions

Step 1

Preheat an outdoor grill for medium heat and lightly oil the grate.

Step 2

Beat the egg and onion together in a mixing bowl. Add the turkey, Italian bread crumbs, liquid smoke, Worcestershire sauce, salt, and pepper. Mix until evenly combined and form into 4 patties. Press each patty into the panko crumbs and set aside.

Step 3

Cook the turkey burgers on the preheated grill until no longer pink in the center and the juices run clear, about 4 minutes per side. An instant-read thermometer inserted into the center should read at least 165 degrees F (74 degrees C). While the burgers are cooking, brush the mushrooms with olive oil and cook on the grill along with the Canadian bacon. Just before the turkey burgers are done, top with the grilled Canadian bacon slices and the Gouda cheese. Cook until the cheese melts.

Step 4

Spread the hamburger buns with mustard and mayonnaise. Place a turkey burger onto each bottom bun and top with the portobello mushroom slices. Sandwich with the remaining bun halves and serve.

Nutrition Facts

Per Serving:

795 calories; protein 44.3g; carbohydrates 41.6g; fat 51g; cholesterol 186.9mg; sodium 1806mg.

Vegan Jicama Ceviche

Recipe Summary

prep: 15 mins

additional: 20 mins

total: 35 mins

Servings: 12

Yield: 12 tostadas

Ingredients

1 large jicama, peeled and grated

1 cup lime juice

2 tablespoons olive oil

2 tablespoons ketchup

1 pound plum tomatoes, seeded and chopped

1 white onion, chopped

¼ cup finely chopped cilantro

1 pinch dried oregano

salt and ground black pepper to taste

12 tostada shells

2 avocados - peeled, pitted, and mashed

Directions

Instructions

Step 1

Combine jicama and lime juice in a large glass bowl and let stand for 20 minutes, stirring every 5 minutes to make sure that all jicama pieces are coated with lime juice. Drain some of the lime juice, depending on your taste.

Step 2

Mix olive oil and ketchup into the jicama. Stir in tomatoes, onion, and cilantro. Season with oregano, salt, and pepper.

Step 3

Serve ceviche on tostadas and garnish with avocado.

Nutrition Facts

Per Serving:

194 calories; protein 3g; carbohydrates 24.9g; fat 10.4g; sodium 100.2mg.

Chicken Stir-Fry with Thai Peanut Sauce

Recipe Summary

prep: 40 mins

cook: 15 mins

total: 55 mins

Servings: 6

Yield: 6 servings

Ingredients

⅔ cup creamy, low-salt peanut butter

1 cup hot water, divided

¼ cup brown sugar

2 tablespoons low-sodium soy sauce

2 tablespoons rice vinegar

1 tablespoon red curry paste, or more to taste

¼ cup canola oil, divided

1 ½ pounds boneless chicken breasts, cut into 1/2-inch cubes

1 tablespoon minced fresh ginger

1 tablespoon minced garlic, or more to taste

1 cup broccoli florets

1 large carrot, cut into thick strips

½ cup halved green beans

½ cup sliced zucchini

1 small onion, sliced

½ sweet red pepper, thinly sliced

3 scallions, sliced

½ cup unsalted, dry-roasted peanuts, divided

½ cup chopped fresh cilantro, divided

1 lime, cut into wedges

1 pinch red pepper flakes, or to taste (Optional)

Directions

Instructions

Step 1

Whisk peanut butter, 1/3 cup hot water, brown sugar, soy sauce, rice vinegar, and curry paste together in a bowl. Set peanut sauce aside.

Step 2

Heat 2 tablespoons oil in a deep skillet or large wok over medium-high heat. Add chicken, ginger, and garlic. Saute, stirring constantly, until chicken is no longer pink in the center and juices run clear, 5 to 7 minutes. Remove chicken from skillet and set aside.

Step 3

Pour 2/3 cup hot water into skillet. Add broccoli, carrot, and green beans. Cover and steam for 2 minutes. Remove vegetables from skillet and reserve steaming liquid in a bowl.

Step 4

Add 1 tablespoon oil to skillet. Add zucchini, onion, and red pepper; stir-fry for 4 minutes. Return steamed broccoli, carrots, and green beans to the skillet. Add remaining oil, if needed. Continue cooking until vegetables are tender but still crisp, 3 to 5 minutes more. Reduce heat to medium-low.

Step 5

Return cooked chicken to skillet. Add peanut sauce, scallions, 1/3 cup peanuts, and 1/3 cup cilantro. Stir thoroughly and heat through, 1 to 3 minutes. Add reserved steaming liquid to thin sauce, if necessary.

Step 6

Garnish with lime wedge and remaining peanuts and cilantro. Sprinkle with red pepper flakes.

Cook's Note:

Use coconut oil in place of canola, if you prefer.

Nutrition Facts

Per Serving:

527 calories; protein 36.4g; carbohydrates 26.4g; fat 34.8g; cholesterol 64.6mg; sodium 307.7mg.

Sesame Cabbage and Mushrooms

Recipe Summary

prep: 15 mins

cook: 6 mins

total: 21 mins

Servings: 4

Yield: 2 cups stir-fry

Ingredients

- 2 ½ tablespoons dark sesame oil, divided
- 6 ounces shiitake mushroom caps, sliced
- 4 cups thinly sliced napa cabbage
- 1 tablespoon reduced-sodium soy sauce
- ¼ teaspoon freshly ground black pepper
- ¼ cup cilantro leaves
- 2 tablespoons toasted sesame seeds

Directions

Instructions

Step 1

Heat a large skillet over high heat. Add 2 tablespoons sesame oil; swirl to coat. Saute mushrooms until browned, about 4 minutes. Add cabbage; saute for 2 minutes.

Step 2

Remove skillet from heat. Mix in 1 1/2 teaspoon sesame oil, soy sauce, and black pepper until well combined. Top with cilantro and sesame seeds.

Nutrition Facts

Per Serving:

133 calories; protein 2.9g; carbohydrates 6.4g; fat 10.9g; sodium 150.9mg.

Vegan-Friendly Falafel

Recipe Summary

prep: 25 mins

additional: 1 day

total: 1 day

Servings: 10

Yield: 30 servings

Ingredients

1 pound dry garbanzo beans

1 onion, quartered

1 potato, peeled and quartered

4 cloves garlic, minced

½ cup cilantro leaves, chopped

1 teaspoon ground coriander

1 teaspoon ground cumin

2 teaspoons salt

½ teaspoon ground black pepper

½ teaspoon cayenne pepper

2 teaspoons fresh lemon juice

1 tablespoon olive oil

1 tablespoon all-purpose flour

2 teaspoons baking soda

2 cups canola oil

Directions

Instructions

Step 1

Rinse the garbanzo beans under cold water and discard any bad ones. Place in a large pot, and cover with water. Let soak 24 hours, and rinse again.

Step 2

Place the garbanzo beans, onion, and potato in the bowl of a food processor. Cover, and process until finely chopped. Leaving about 1 cup of the garbanzo bean mixture in the food processor bowl, pour the rest into a mixing bowl. Add the garlic, cilantro, coriander, cumin, salt, pepper, and cayenne pepper to the garbanzo bean mixture in the food processor bowl; process on low to blend thoroughly. Return the reserved garbanzo bean mixture to the food processor bowl, and add the lemon juice, olive oil, and flour; process on low into a coarse meal. Cover, and refrigerate 2 hours.

Step 3

Stir the baking soda into the garbanzo bean mixture until evenly blended. Using damp hands, form the mixture into 1 1/2 inch diameter balls.

Step 4

Pour the canola oil into a wok 1 to 2 inches deep, and heat over medium-high heat. Cook the falafel balls, turning so all sides are evenly browned, about 5 minutes. Remove falafel from oil, and drain on paper towels. Repeat to cook remaining falafel balls.

Cook's Tip

If you don't have time to soak the dry garbanzo beans for this recipe, substitute three 15 ounce cans of garbanzo beans, and start with Step 2.

Nutrition Facts

Per Serving:

245 calories; protein 9.6g; carbohydrates 33.8g; fat 8.7g; sodium 731.2mg.

Korean Soft Tofu Stew (Soon Du Bu Jigae)

Recipe Summary

prep: 5 mins

cook: 15 mins

total: 20 mins

Servings: 2

Yield: 2 servings

Ingredients

1 teaspoon vegetable oil

1 teaspoon Korean chile powder

2 tablespoons ground beef (Optional)

1 tablespoon Korean soy bean paste (doenjang)

1 cup water

salt and pepper to taste

1 (12 ounce) package Korean soon tofu or soft tofu, drained and sliced

1 egg

1 teaspoon sesame seeds

1 green onion, chopped

Directions

Instructions

Step 1

Heat the vegetable oil in a large saucepan over medium heat. Stir in the Korean chile powder and ground beef. Cook and stir until the beef is crumbly, evenly browned, and no longer pink. Stir in the soy bean paste, coating the beef. Pour in the water and bring to a boil. Season with salt and pepper. Gently drop tofu into the soup and continue cooking until the tofu is heated through, 1 to 2 minutes. Remove from heat and quickly add the egg into the soup, stirring gently to break it up. Garnish with sesame seeds and green onion.

Nutrition Facts

Per Serving:

242 calories; protein 20g; carbohydrates 7g; fat 16.5g; cholesterol 99.4mg; sodium 415.1mg.

Aloo Gobi

Recipe Summary

prep: 30 mins

cook: 35 mins

total: 1 hr 5 mins

Servings: 6

Yield: 6 servings

Ingredients

3 tablespoons vegetable oil, divided

½ teaspoon cumin seed

1 small onion, quartered and sliced

2 serrano chile peppers, minced

1 teaspoon ginger paste

2 teaspoons ground coriander

¼ teaspoon paprika

½ teaspoon turmeric powder

½ teaspoon cayenne pepper

½ teaspoon garam masala

2 medium baking potatoes, peeled and cut into 1 inch pieces

1 teaspoon salt

½ head cauliflower, cut into florets

2 teaspoons lemon juice

Directions

Instructions

Step 1

Heat 2 tablespoons of oil over medium-high heat in a large pot. Fry cumin seeds for a few seconds until they turn golden brown and begin to pop. Reduce heat to medium, stir in the onion, and cook until lightly browned. Stir in serrano pepper and ginger; fry for 1 minute. Season with coriander, paprika, turmeric, cayenne, and garam masala; cook for 30 seconds until fragrant.

Step 2

Stir potatoes and salt into the pot, cover, and cook for 5 to 7 minutes. Add cauliflower, cover, and cook until cauliflower steams in its own juices until tender, about 20 minutes. Stir in lemon juice. Pour remaining 1 tablespoon of oil around the edges of the pot. Increase heat to medium-high and fry for 3 to 5 minutes to brown, stirring gently to avoid mashing the cauliflower.

Nutrition Facts

Per Serving:

141 calories; protein 2.8g; carbohydrates 17.8g; fat 7.3g; sodium 408.2mg.

Grilled Pesto Chicken Kabobs

Recipe Summary

prep: 20 mins

cook: 10 mins

additional: 4 hrs

total: 4 hrs 30 mins

Servings: 6

Yield: 6 servings

Ingredients

Marinade:

¼ cup vegetable oil

2 tablespoons cooking sherry

2 tablespoons prepared pesto

1 tablespoon freshly squeezed lemon juice

½ teaspoon salt

¼ teaspoon pepper

Kabobs:

1 ½ pounds boneless skinless chicken breasts, cut into 1-inch chunks

1 (8 ounce) package mushrooms

1 small zucchini, cut into chunks

1 medium red onion, cut into chunks

12 grape tomatoes

6 metal skewers

Directions

Instructions

Step 1

Whisk oil, sherry, pesto, lemon juice, salt, and pepper together in a glass bowl. Add chicken pieces and stir to coat. Cover and refrigerate for 4 hours to overnight.

Step 2

Preheat an outdoor grill for medium-high heat and lightly oil the grate.

Step 3

Thread marinated chicken, mushrooms, zucchini, red onion, and tomatoes alternately onto skewers. Reserve remaining marinade.

Step 4

Place kabobs onto the preheated grill, and cook, turning occasionally and brushing with the reserved marinade, until chicken is cooked and juices run clear, 10 to 15 minutes.

Cook's Note:

If you're using wooden skewers, soak them in water for 20 minutes prior to use.

Nutrition Facts

Per Serving:

263 calories; protein 26.4g; carbohydrates 6.4g; fat 14.5g; cholesterol 66.3mg; sodium 327.3mg.

Spicy Honey-Lime Chicken Thigh Kebabs

Recipe Summary

prep: 20 mins

cook: 15 mins

total: 35 mins

Servings: 4

Yield: 4 servings

Ingredients

Glaze:

¼ cup honey

2 tablespoons Sriracha sauce

1 tablespoon lime juice

Kebabs:

8 large metal skewers

1 pound skinless, boneless chicken thighs, cut into 1 1/2-inch pieces

1 red sweet pepper, cut into 1 1/2-inch pieces

1 medium zucchini, cut into 1 1/2-inch pieces

½ small fresh pineapple, cored and cut into 1 1/2-inch pieces

1 medium red onion, cut into 1 1/2-inch chunks

2 tablespoons olive oil

salt and freshly ground black pepper to taste

1 pinch garlic powder, or more to taste

1 teaspoon lime zest (Optional)

Directions

Instructions

Step 1

Preheat an outdoor grill for medium-high heat and lightly oil the grate.

Step 2

Whisk honey, Sriracha sauce, and lime juice together in a small bowl. Set aside.

Step 3

Thread chicken, red pepper, zucchini, pineapple, and red onion alternately onto skewers and place on a platter. Brush with olive oil, then season with salt, pepper, and garlic powder.

Step 4

Arrange skewers on the hot grate. Close lid and reduce heat to medium. Grill until chicken is cooked through, turning skewers every few minutes, 15 to 20 minutes. Brush glaze on all sides of skewers during the last 2 to 3 minutes, turning to lightly caramelize glaze. Transfer to a serving platter and grate lime zest on top. Serve warm.

Nutrition Facts

Per Serving:

360 calories; protein 20.5g; carbohydrates 28.7g; fat 18.7g; cholesterol 70.4mg; sodium 428.5mg.

Instant Pot® Egg Roll in a Bowl

Recipe Summary

prep: 15 mins

cook: 30 mins

total: 45 mins

Servings: 4

Yield: 4 servings

Ingredients

2 tablespoons olive oil

½ cup diced sweet onion

½ cup grated carrot

1 teaspoon minced garlic

½ pound ground chicken

½ cup bulk pork sausage

4 ½ cups sliced cabbage

½ cup water

2 tablespoons tamari

1 tablespoon honey

½ teaspoon ground ginger

½ teaspoon freshly ground black pepper

¼ teaspoon salt

1 teaspoon sesame oil (Optional)

Directions

Instructions

Step 1

Turn on a multi-functional pressure cooker (such as Instant Pot®) and select Saute function. Add olive oil, followed by onion, carrot, and garlic; cook until onion is translucent, 5 to 7 minutes. Add ground chicken and ground sausage and cook until browned, 5 to 10 minutes.

Step 2

Stir in cabbage, water, tamari, honey, ginger, pepper, and salt. Close and lock the lid. Select high pressure according to manufacturer's instructions; set timer for 10 minutes. Allow 10 to 15 minutes for pressure to build.

Step 3

Release pressure using the natural-release method according to manufacturer's instructions, 10 to 15 minutes. Stir and add sesame oil.

Cook's Note:

You can use brown sugar instead of honey if you like.

Nutrition Facts

Per Serving:

232 calories; protein 17.7g; carbohydrates 14.6g; fat 11.9g; cholesterol 41mg; sodium 841mg.

Danish Cinnamon Snails

Recipe Summary

prep: 1 hr

cook: 10 mins

additional: 30 mins

total: 1 hr 40 mins

Servings: 15

Yield: 15 rolls

Ingredients

Dough:

1 cup warm milk (110 degrees F/45 degrees C)

3 (0.6 ounce) cakes cake yeast

6 ½ tablespoons butter, room temperature

2 eggs

½ teaspoon ground cardamom

2 tablespoons white sugar

¼ teaspoon salt

4 cups all-purpose flour, or as needed

Filling:

⅔ cup butter, softened

½ cup white sugar

2 tablespoons ground cinnamon

Directions

Instructions

Step 1

Pour the warm milk into a mixing bowl and mash in the fresh cake yeast. Mix in 6 1/2 tablespoons of soft butter, eggs, cardamom, 2 tablespoons sugar, salt, and 3

1/2 cups of the flour. Use a wooden spoon to mix the dough. If it's very sticky, mix in the remaining 1/2 cup of flour. Cover the bowl and let the dough rise for 30 minutes.

Step 2

Cream together the 2/3 cup butter and 1/2 cup sugar. Stir in the cinnamon.

Step 3

Transfer the dough to a floured surface and knead it until it's firm, about 3 minutes. Divide the dough in half; roll each half into a rectangle no more than 1/2 inch thick. Spread each rectangle with half the filling.

Step 4

Stack one layer of dough and filling on top of the other rectangle of dough, filling-side up. Roll the dough up, starting with the edge closest to you, to form a long log. Cut the log into 1 inch-thick slices.

Step 5

Preheat an oven to 425 degrees F (220 degrees C). Line a baking sheet with parchment paper, or grease a baking dish or two cake pans.

Step 6

Place the rolls on the prepared baking sheet, spacing them about 3 inches apart. If you like pull-apart rolls, arrange them in a greased baking dish or cake pans, spacing the rolls about 1 inch apart. Place the uneven end pieces on the baking sheet cut-side up for the best presentation. Let the rolls rest 20 minutes before baking.

Step 7

Bake the snails in the preheated oven until golden brown, about 10 minutes. Pull-apart rolls will take longer to bake: after 10 minutes, reduce the oven temperature to 350 degrees F (175 degrees C) and bake the rolls until the sides are fully set, about 10 minutes longer. Cover the baking dish with foil if the rolls begin to get too brown.

Nutrition Facts

Per Serving:

301 calories; protein 6.3g; carbohydrates 36.7g; fat 14.6g; cholesterol 58mg; sodium 148mg.

Asian Lettuce Wraps

Recipe Summary

prep: 20 mins

cook: 15 mins

total: 35 mins

Servings: 4

Yield: 4 servings

Ingredients

16 Boston Bibb or butter lettuce leaves

1 pound lean ground beef

1 tablespoon cooking oil

1 large onion, chopped

¼ cup hoisin sauce

2 cloves fresh garlic, minced

1 tablespoon soy sauce

1 tablespoon rice wine vinegar

2 teaspoons minced pickled ginger

1 dash Asian chile pepper sauce, or to taste (Optional)

1 (8 ounce) can water chestnuts, drained and finely chopped

1 bunch green onions, chopped

2 teaspoons Asian (dark) sesame oil

Directions

Instructions

Step 1

Rinse whole lettuce leaves and pat dry, being careful not tear them. Set aside.

Step 2

Heat a large skillet over medium-high heat. Cook and stir beef and cooking oil in the hot skillet until browned and crumbly, 5 to 7 minutes. Drain and discard grease; transfer beef to a bowl. Cook and stir onion in the same skillet used for beef until slightly tender, 5 to 10 minutes. Stir hoisin sauce, garlic, soy sauce, vinegar, ginger, and chile pepper sauce into onions. Add water chestnuts, green onions, sesame oil, and cooked beef; cook and stir until the onions just begin to wilt, about 2 minutes.

Step 3

Arrange lettuce leaves around the outer edge of a large serving platter and pile meat mixture in the center.

Nutrition Facts

Per Serving:

388 calories; protein 23.4g; carbohydrates 24.3g; fat 22.3g; cholesterol 68.9mg; sodium 579.6mg.

Chicken Stir-Fry with Thai Peanut Sauce

Recipe Summary

prep: 40 mins

cook: 15 mins

total: 55 mins

Servings: 6

Yield: 6 servings

Ingredients

⅔ cup creamy, low-salt peanut butter

1 cup hot water, divided

¼ cup brown sugar

2 tablespoons low-sodium soy sauce

2 tablespoons rice vinegar

1 tablespoon red curry paste, or more to taste

¼ cup canola oil, divided

1 ½ pounds boneless chicken breasts, cut into 1/2-inch cubes

1 tablespoon minced fresh ginger

1 tablespoon minced garlic, or more to taste

1 cup broccoli florets

1 large carrot, cut into thick strips

½ cup halved green beans

½ cup sliced zucchini

1 small onion, sliced

½ sweet red pepper, thinly sliced

3 scallions, sliced

½ cup unsalted, dry-roasted peanuts, divided

½ cup chopped fresh cilantro, divided

1 lime, cut into wedges

1 pinch red pepper flakes, or to taste (Optional)

Directions

Instructions

Step 1

Whisk peanut butter, 1/3 cup hot water, brown sugar, soy sauce, rice vinegar, and curry paste together in a bowl. Set peanut sauce aside.

Step 2

Heat 2 tablespoons oil in a deep skillet or large wok over medium-high heat. Add chicken, ginger, and garlic. Saute, stirring constantly, until chicken is no longer pink in the center and juices run clear, 5 to 7 minutes. Remove chicken from skillet and set aside.

Step 3

Pour 2/3 cup hot water into skillet. Add broccoli, carrot, and green beans. Cover and steam for 2 minutes. Remove vegetables from skillet and reserve steaming liquid in a bowl.

Step 4

Add 1 tablespoon oil to skillet. Add zucchini, onion, and red pepper; stir-fry for 4 minutes. Return steamed broccoli, carrots, and green beans to the skillet. Add remaining oil, if needed. Continue cooking until vegetables are tender but still crisp, 3 to 5 minutes more. Reduce heat to medium-low.

Step 5

Return cooked chicken to skillet. Add peanut sauce, scallions, 1/3 cup peanuts, and 1/3 cup cilantro. Stir thoroughly and heat through, 1 to 3 minutes. Add reserved steaming liquid to thin sauce, if necessary.

Step 6

Garnish with lime wedge and remaining peanuts and cilantro. Sprinkle with red pepper flakes.

Cook's Note:

Use coconut oil in place of canola, if you prefer.

Nutrition Facts

Per Serving:

527 calories; protein 36.4g; carbohydrates 26.4g; fat 34.8g; cholesterol 64.6mg; sodium 307.7mg.

Pancetta Wrapped Shrimp with Chipotle Vinaigrette and Cilantro Oil

Recipe Summary

prep: 30 mins

cook: 10 mins

total: 40 mins

Servings: 8

Yield: 8 servings

Ingredients

1 bunch cilantro, rinsed

1 cup canola oil

1 teaspoon honey

4 teaspoons fresh lime juice

Salt to taste

1 canned chipotle pepper

1 tablespoon adobo sauce from canned chipotle peppers

¼ cup fresh lemon juice

½ cup rice vinegar

1 clove garlic

1 cup canola oil

Salt to taste

3 pounds extra large shrimp (16-20), peeled and deveined, tail left on

2 pounds thinly sliced pancetta

Directions

Instructions

Step 1

Prepare cilantro oil by pureeing cilantro, canola oil, honey, lime juice, and salt to taste until smooth; pour into a bowl or bottle, and set aside.

Step 2

Prepare the chipotle vinaigrette by pureeing the chipotle pepper, adobo sauce, lemon juice, rice vinegar, and garlic in a blender until smooth. With the blender running, slowly pour in the canola oil, and puree until creamy. Season to taste with salt, and set aside.

Step 3

Preheat a grill for medium heat.

Step 4

Cut the pancetta slices in half. Wrap a half slice of pancetta around each shrimp to cover. Grill until the pancetta has crisped, and the shrimp has turned opaque, 2 to 3 minutes per side. Drain on paper towels.

Step 5

To serve, arrange cooked shrimp on a warmed serving platter or individual plates, and drizzle with chipotle vinaigrette and cilantro oil.

Nutrition Facts

Per Serving:

839 calories; protein 41.9g; carbohydrates 2.8g; fat 73.2g; cholesterol 300.5mg; sodium 1183.2mg.

Spicy Mexican Tuna Salad

Recipe Summary

prep: 10 mins

total: 10 mins

Servings: 8

Yield: 8 servings

Ingredients

1 (5 ounce) can tuna, drained

1 cup frozen peas, thawed and drained

2 chipotle peppers in adobo sauce, or more to taste - chopped

1 tablespoon mayonnaise, or to taste

¼ teaspoon dried minced onion, or to taste

1 pinch garlic salt, or to taste

1 pinch ground black pepper, or to taste

Directions

Instructions

Step 1

Mix tuna, peas, chipotle peppers, mayonnaise, dried minced onion, garlic salt, and black pepper in a bowl until thoroughly combined.

Nutrition Facts

Per Serving:

47 calories; protein 5g; carbohydrates 3g; fat 1.6g; cholesterol 5.4mg; sodium 95.9mg.

Grilled Fish Tacos with Chipotle-Lime Dressing

Recipe Summary

prep: 35 mins

cook: 9 mins

additional: 6 hrs

total: 6 hrs 44 mins

Servings: 6

Yield: 6 servings

Ingredients

Marinade

¼ cup extra virgin olive oil

2 tablespoons distilled white vinegar

2 tablespoons fresh lime juice

2 teaspoons lime zest

1 ½ teaspoons honey

2 cloves garlic, minced

½ teaspoon cumin

½ teaspoon chili powder

1 teaspoon seafood seasoning, such as Old Bay™

½ teaspoon ground black pepper

1 teaspoon hot pepper sauce, or to taste

1 pound tilapia fillets, cut into chunks

Dressing

1 (8 ounce) container light sour cream

½ cup adobo sauce from chipotle peppers

2 tablespoons fresh lime juice

2 teaspoons lime zest

¼ teaspoon cumin

¼ teaspoon chili powder

½ teaspoon seafood seasoning, such as Old Bay™

salt and pepper to taste

Toppings

1 (10 ounce) package tortillas

3 ripe tomatoes, seeded and diced

1 bunch cilantro, chopped

1 small head cabbage, cored and shredded

2 limes, cut in wedges

Directions

Instructions

Step 1

To make the marinade, whisk together the olive oil, vinegar, lime juice, lime zest, honey, garlic, cumin, chili powder, seafood seasoning, black pepper, and hot sauce in a bowl until blended. Place the tilapia in a shallow dish, and pour the marinade over the fish. Cover, and refrigerate 6 to 8 hours.

Step 2

To make the dressing, combine the sour cream and adobo sauce in a bowl. Stir in the lime juice, lime zest, cumin, chili powder, seafood seasoning. Add salt, and pepper in desired amounts. Cover, and refrigerate until needed.

Step 3

Preheat an outdoor grill for high heat and lightly oil grate. Set grate 4 inches from the heat.

Step 4

Remove fish from marinade, drain off any excess and discard marinade. Grill fish pieces until easily flaked with a fork, turning once, about 9 minutes.

Step 5

Assemble tacos by placing fish pieces in the center of tortillas with desired amounts of tomatoes, cilantro, and cabbage; drizzle with dressing. To serve, roll up tortillas around fillings, and garnish with lime wedges.

Cook's Note:

The marinated fish in this recipe can also be cooked in the oven. Preheat oven to 350 degrees F (175 degrees C). Bake fish in preheated oven until it easily flakes with a fork, 9 to 11 minutes. Assemble tacos according to directions. Mahi-mahi can be substituted for the tilapia.

Nutrition Facts

Per Serving:

416 calories; protein 22.6g; carbohydrates 38.5g; fat 19.2g; cholesterol 42.6mg; sodium 644.3mg.

Fish Tacos with Honey-Cumin Cilantro Slaw and Chipotle Mayo

Recipe Summary

prep: 30 mins

cook: 10 mins

additional: 4 hrs

total: 4 hrs 40 mins

Servings: 4

Yield: 8 tacos

Ingredients

1 pound tilapia fillets, cut into chunks

½ cup fresh lime juice

⅓ cup fresh lime juice

2 tablespoons honey

1 tablespoon vegetable oil

1 teaspoon ground cumin

½ cup mayonnaise

2 chipotle chilies in adobo sauce

1 tablespoon adobo sauce from chipotle peppers

¼ teaspoon salt

⅛ teaspoon cayenne pepper

⅓ cup all-purpose flour

2 eggs, lightly beaten

2 cups panko crumbs

salt and ground black pepper to taste

1 cup vegetable oil for frying

2 cups 3 color coleslaw blend

1 cup minced fresh cilantro leaves

8 (7 inch) flour tortillas, warmed

Directions

Instructions

Step 1

Place the tilapia chunks in a flat dish and pour 1/2 cup lime juice over the fish. Cover, and refrigerate at least 4 hours.

Step 2

Meanwhile, make the honey-cumin sauce by whisking together 1/3 cup lime juice, honey, vegetable oil, and ground cumin a small bowl. Set aside until needed.

Step 3

To make the chipotle mayonnaise dressing, place the mayonnaise, chilies, adobo sauce, 1/4 teaspoon salt, and cayenne pepper together in the bowl of a food processor. Pulse until smooth. Cover, and refrigerate until needed.

Step 4

To bread the fish, place the flour, eggs, and panko crumbs in three separate shallow dishes. Season the fish with salt and pepper to taste. Dip the fish pieces first in the four, coating evenly, and shaking off any excess. Dip next in the eggs, and last in the panko crumbs, patting the pieces to help the breadcrumbs hold. Set the fish aside on a plate.

Step 5

To cook the breaded fish, pour 1 cup vegetable oil into a skillet to 1/4 inch deep. Heat the oil to 365 degrees F (185 degrees C) over medium heat. Cook the fish, turning until all sides are golden brown, and flesh is easily flaked with a fork. Drain on paper towels. Brush the fish with the honey-cumin sauce.

Step 6

Mix the coleslaw and cilantro together in a bowl. Reserve 1/4 cup of the chipotle mayonnaise dressing, and pour the remaining dressing over the coleslaw mixture. Toss to coat evenly with the dressing.

Step 7

Place the tortillas on a flat surface, and spread each with 1 tablespoon reserved chipotle mayonnaise dressing. Divide the fish between the tortillas. Top with the cilantro coleslaw.

Tips

The nutrition data for this recipe includes the full amount of the breading ingredients. The actual amount of the breading consumed will vary. We have determined the nutritional value of oil for frying based on a retention value of 10% after cooking. The exact amount will vary depending on cooking time and temperature, ingredient density, and the specific type of oil used.

Nutrition Facts

Per Serving:

984 calories; protein 42.2g; carbohydrates 117.5g; fat 44.4g; cholesterol 137.4mg; sodium 1153.8mg.

Million-Dollar Spaghetti

Recipe Summary

prep: 25 mins

cook: 1 hr 5 mins

total: 1 hr 30 mins

Servings: 8

Yield: 8 servings

Ingredients

1 (8 ounce) package spaghetti

1 pound lean ground beef

1 (16 ounce) jar spaghetti sauce

½ cup butter, sliced - divided

1 (8 ounce) container cottage cheese

1 (8 ounce) package cream cheese, softened

¼ cup sour cream

1 (8 ounce) package shredded sharp Cheddar cheese

Directions

Instructions

Step 1

Preheat oven to 350 degrees F (175 degrees C).

Step 2

Bring a large pot of lightly salted water to a boil. Cook spaghetti in the boiling water, stirring occasionally until cooked through but firm to the bite, about 12 minutes. Drain.

Step 3

Heat a large skillet over medium-high heat. Cook and stir beef in the hot skillet until browned and crumbly, 5 to 7 minutes; drain and discard grease. Transfer to a bowl and mix spaghetti sauce into ground beef.

Step 4

Place half the slices of butter into the bottom of a 9x13-inch casserole dish. Spread half the spaghetti into the dish. Mix cottage cheese, cream cheese, and sour cream together in a bowl; spread mixture over spaghetti. Layer remaining spaghetti over creamy mixture. Top with remaining pats of butter.

Step 5

Pour ground beef mixture over spaghetti and spread to cover casserole.

Step 6

Bake in the preheated oven for 30 minutes. Spread Cheddar cheese over casserole and continue baking until cheese has melted and is lightly browned, about 15 more minutes.

Nutrition Facts

Per Serving:

618 calories; protein 28.4g; carbohydrates 30.8g; fat 42.2g; cholesterol 136.4mg; sodium 721mg.

Easy Shrimp Ceviche

Recipe Summary

prep: 15 mins

cook: 5 mins

additional: 20 mins

total: 40 mins

Servings: 4

Yield: 4 servings

Ingredients

1 cucumber, diced

2 Roma tomatoes, diced

½ medium red onion, diced

2 serrano peppers, seeded and deveined

¼ cup chopped cilantro

6 medium limes, divided

1 ½ teaspoons salt, divided

½ teaspoon ground black pepper to taste

½ pound raw shrimp, peeled and deveined

1 small avocado, diced (Optional)

Directions

Instructions

Step 1

Combine cucumber, tomatoes, red onion, serrano peppers, and cilantro in a bowl. Add 1 teaspoon salt and squeeze 1 lime. Gently mix and set aside.

Step 2

Squeeze the remaining limes into another bowl. Add remaining salt and pepper.

Step 3

Bring a 1- to 2-quart pot of water to a boil. Place shrimp into the boiling water for 45 seconds. Quickly remove from the water using a strainer.

Step 4

Chop the partially cooked shrimp into small pieces and add to the bowl with the seasoned lime mixture. Let sit for 20 minutes. Combine with the cucumber mixture and top with avocados.

Cook's Note:

Unlike fish ceviche recipes, shrimp should not marinade in lime/lemon juice for hours. The poaching technique will give the shrimp a stable texture and also minimize the risks associated with consuming raw seafood.

Nutrition Facts

Per Serving:

163 calories; protein 11.7g; carbohydrates 19g; fat 7.1g; cholesterol 86.3mg; sodium 981mg.

www.ingramcontent.com/pod-product-compliance
Ingram Content Group UK Ltd.
Pitfield, Milton Keynes, MK11 3LW, UK
UKHW021934200726
13853UKWH00011B/1881